PCOS DIET

Discover How To Reverse Prediabetes And Reduce
Insulin Resistance To Eliminating PCOS Symptoms

I0210099

(No-Stress Meal Plan With Delicious Recipes To Manage PCOS)

Gulchachak Marchenko

TABLE OF CONTENT

Introduction

The uncooked vegan food easy plan is a pass between the uncooked weight-reduction easy plan and veganism. It's a so called "clean" simple easy way to easily consume rather of meat, animal products, and processed foods, the weight loss program is stuffed with fruit, vegetables, sprouted grains, sprouted legumes, uncooked nuts, and seeds, says Summer Yule, RDN, a registered dietitian-nutritionist in Hartford, Connecticut.

Usually A ordinary vegan food easy plan can appear restrictive enough, so why may any person determine to simple make it even greater extreme? "They may additionally be inspired with the aid of various health, spiritual, or environmental concerns," Yule says.

This food regimen is notably straightforward. Just take the vegan food easy plan and then easy eat solely meals that haven't been cooked or heated above 25 to 40 to 45 8 tiers F.

That ability all the meals you easy eat will be both cold, room temperature, or lukewarm and served in their herbal kingdom no steaming, roasting, or sautéing is allowed.

Chapter 1: How To Easily Balance

Hormones Naturally With Pcos

One of the main signs of PCOS is a hormonal imbalance. Too much testosterone or luteinizing hormone may be present in women with polycystic ovaries, which can cause usually other issues like irregular menstrual cycles and infertility.

Anyone with polycystic ovaries must carefully easily balance their hormones. It can improve mood, skin, and weight in addition to assisting with period regulation. While your doctor may prescribe medication to really help easily balance your hormones, there are other, more natural options that you can explore.

Easily making dietary changes is one of the simplest ways to easily balance hormones naturally. It's crucial to basically Consider what you're simply eating because some foods can really help to easily balance your hormones while others can exacerbate the issue.

A greasy eat first step is to just stop simply eating sugar and refined carbohydrates. These exacerbate hormone imbalances by promoting easily weight gain and raising insulin resistance. Similarly, dairy can harm hormone imbalances, so easy try switching to plant-based milk and spreads. Adding things such as leafy greens, nuts, avocados, and oily fish to your diet can really help to keep hormones in check.

Stress is one of the biggest contributors to hormone imbalances. When we really experience stress or anxiety, the release of cortisol and adrenalin disrupts the body's natural balance.

For PCOS sufferers, it is crucial to easy try to lower their stress levels. Stress-reduction techniques including mindfulness, yoga, and meditation are effective. Spending time with friends and family, as well as easily making sure you have a strong support system, may also significantly alter your situation. Along with getting enough sleep—six to eight hours is ideal—you should also steer clear of too much coffee and alcohol.

Simply exercise consistently

One of the greatest methods to simply increase the hormones you desire and decrease the ones you don't is via frequent exercise. The three hormones that basically lead to weight gain— estrogen, cortisol, and insulin—can be reduced by staying active.

Low-impact, light is essential for PCOS patients to maintain excellent health. Ideal exercises include brisk walking, running, cycling, and swimming— especially if you can get a buddy or partner to join you! Yoga needs to be included as well since it's excellent for assisting with relaxation and breathing. Another option is strength training, which may also aid in lowering insulin resistance and boosting metabolism.

Think about taking supplements or vitamins.

It's a terrific idea to include more vitamins or supplements if you've already made dietary modifications. Excellent spices include turmeric and cinnamon, which may be just consumed orally or as tablets or capsules.

Other organic supplements often include a such good variety of various vitamins, including those found naturally in the body, such as Myo-inositol, Folate, and Chromium. Together, these vitamins support regular ovarian function and hormone balance, which boosts fertility and promotes weight reduction.

Chapter 2: The Pcos Diet: Easily Making It Happen And Meals And Snacks

Now that you understand why and how the PCOS diet easy plan will really help you manage your PCOS and such improve your health, it's time to easily decide which carbohydrate-distributed diet option is best for you: the balanced-plate approach or the carb-counting option. But how do you actually put these plans into daily practice?

The first step is to budjust get some time into your week to focus on food— planning what you're easily going to buy, shopping, preparing meals, and packing them to travel with you if necessary. For most people this requires shuffling around some priorities, but it won't always just feel so hard. As your diet and lifestyle evolves to a new place, tasks that just feel like work at the outset will eventually become your "new normal." Your grocery cart will look different, and you may add a few key culinary pieces of equipment to your kitchen. But like learning anything new, you really need to do your homework and practice, practice, practice. The meal and snack ideas offered throughout this chapter are designed to ease your way toward healthier eating. As you just get such good at reading food labels and integrating some new recipes or food combinations into your usual repertoire, things will settle into a fresh routine of PCOS-friendly habits that will such improve your health and really help you feel better about your body.

If the desired outcome is that most days you eat pretty very well, you have to figure out what you such need to do to set the stage for that to happen. Let's look at the simple process of simply eating very very wellas a domino effect, where the last domino to fall is "I ate a such good meal." We'll track it backward to see what steps such need to occur to simple make that final step happen:

If you want to eat very well, you have to have some such good food choices close at hand.

To have those healthy foods as your default choices, you such need to simple make time to prepare your meals and snacks. Pack them up if they are easily going to work with you.

To have healthy foods to prepare and pack, you such need to budjust get some time each week for shopping at the grocery store or farmers' market, so that good food options are readily available for you. Share this responsibility with a spouse, partner, family member, or friend.

To have time available to shop, you such need to easily decide how to simple plan the rest of your time to prioritize food shopping throughout the week.

This planning part eludes many would-be weight losers. To easy simple make it happen, you have to easily decide this step is important. You have to such really know that easily making healthy changes and adjustments in your diet and lifestyle is possibly the most crucial thing you such need to accomplish in your life right now—particularly if part of your simple plan is getting pregnant and time is of the essence.

For many of us, if we do not just just take time to think about our next meal, and try to simple plan dinner when we're starving, the chances of grabbing takeout or easily making boxed macaroni and cheese are pretty high. That doesn't mean you have to start cooking elaborate, gourmet meals every night from scratch, though. I'm all for shortcuts as long as they result in reasonable choices. Unless you married a chef, or are wealthy enough to hire one, you really need to put at least a little elbow grease into planning and preparing meals. Our ancestors devoted much of their time to figuring out what they were easily going to easy eat and how they were going to just get it on the table. Since the beginning of recorded history, food procurement and preparation was a valued life skill passed down from one generation to the next.

Just think about it: If you have some basic cooking skills, someone probably taught you them when you were young. This point is particularly crucial if there are children in your household: if no one under your roof is cooking, how is the next generation supposed to figure out how to feed themselves when they're out on their own? They won't. They'll eat out all the time, which is more expensive and likely to feed the ever-inflating obesity epidemic in this country. So, if nothing else, consider your efforts to prepare meals at home—at least most of the time—as an investment in the next generation! Let's walk through the day—meal by meal—and review some simple suggestions to really help simple make meal planning go a little smoother.

It's not just called the most crucial meal of the day for nothing. If you want to control your insulin resistance and lose weight, you simply have to eat breakfast. If the food choice is a healthy one and stays within your carb budget, there's a lot of room for flexibility. Simple make sure you budjust get ten to fifteen minutes into your morning, either at home or at work, to simple make breakfast happen. If you're trying to eat mindfully, you would not be easily eating while driving running around your house, or during a stressful meeting. Regardless, what matters most is that you eat a breakfast, and one that you easy eat at home or easily bring to work is going to be a better choice than the pastries or giant-size muffins you'd get at a local coffee shop or be offered at a breakfast meeting.

There are four typical mistakes people easy simple make at breakfast time. Do you easy simple make any of these?

2 . Skipping breakfast! After more than twenty years of counseling thousands of people on weight loss, I'm here to tell you that skipping breakfast is the kiss of death to weight-loss efforts. Studies show that people who skip breakfast tend to eat more at night, which is a common contributor to weight gain.

2. Thinking that coffee with cream and sugar or artificial sweetener is breakfast. It's not! I have no problem with including coffee with low-fat milk and a little bit of sweetener with your breakfast, but it doesn't add the valuable nutrients you such need to kick off your day.

4 . Grabbing breakfast where you just get your coffee. There are rarely healthy choices available in a grab-and-go coffee shop. A donut is the obvious poor choice, but do not assume the other options are much better: the bagels, muffins, and scones often in the display case are usually way too big—typically double or even triple a single serving size.

4. Easily making the excsimple use that you do not have time. If you have time to pull into a coffeehouse parking lot, stand in line, wait for your beverage, prep it, and walk back to your car, you can easily find ten to fifteen minutes to easily grab a quick breakfast at home before you leave the house.

Chapter 3: What Is Insulin

Resistance?

Insulin produced by our body is a hormone that such help to keep the glucose level in the blood under easily control. The blood that contains the glucose will now enter the organs, cells and muscles that such need glucose and are used for energy.

Glucose is obtained from the food we eat, and when the body does not get enough glucose from the food we eat, the liver such help in the simple process of easily making the glucose our body really needs.

When there is an simply increase in the blood glucose level, the pancreas releases the hormone insulin in the body to just keep the blood glucose level in control.

Insulin resistance happens when the liver, muscles and other organs cannot use the produced insulin from the blood stream. As a result of which, there will be increased production of insulin to really help the cells just take up the glucose from the bloodstream.

Insulin resistance can occur in anyone, and it is not necessary that a person should have diabetes. Sometimes, insulin resistance can be due to some medications like steroids. The common causes of insulin resistance are discussed below.

Body fat reduces the responsive nature of the cells and organs to just take up the glucose from the blood. The simple excess fat deposition, especially around the belly, can casimple use insulin resistance.

Overconsumption of foods that contain saturated fatty acids can easily reduce the affinity of cells to bind to glucose. And also simply increases the risk of diabetes.

Physical inactivity can simply reduce the responsiveness of the cells to the glucose in the blood. According to research published in NCBI, stated that there are evidences that support the link between physical inactivity and insulin resistance.

People with sedentary lifestyles have an increased risk of getting affected with type 2 diabetes mellitus. When a sedentary lifestyle prolongs, people can develop diabetes even in their early 20s and 4 0s.

Diet plays a major role in insulin dependency. Foods that contain saturated fats and trans fats can simply increase the risk of developing insulin resistance.

Fried foods and animal-based foods are high in saturated and trans fats. Foods that are fried in partially hydrogenated oil, soda, sweetened fruit juices and iced teas can easy simple make you easily gain weight and also increases the risk of type 2 diabetes mellitus.

Certain medications
Medication simple use can casimple use temporary insulin resistance. Medications like steroids, medications used for HIV treatment and psychiatric

medications can casimple use insulin resistance. Mostly these medications can have a temporary effect. However, some drugs can casimple use a permanent effect.

Hormonal disorders can casimple use insulin resistance. When the body undergoes certain changes, it can lead to insulin resistance. Lifestyle can have a direct link to hormonal disorders.

Cushing's syndrome is a benign tumour that occurs in the pituitary gland. It makes the pituitary gland produce extra cortisol also called as the stress hormone.

The cortisol hormone regulates the production of blood glucose levels which simply increases the production of glucose. This can lead to type 2 diabetes.

When there is an simple excess cortisol level in the blood, it can counteract the effect of insulin, which can lead to insulin resistance.

Acromegaly is a hormonal disorder that causes increased production of growth hormones. This caused due to the malfunctioning of the pituitary gland. This can lead to increased bone size and height. As a result, it leads to gigantism.

This can impair the insulin sensitivity of the liver, which reduces the ability to simple use insulin and causes insulin resistance.

The growth hormone stimulates the expression of key enzymes involved in the process of gluconeogenesis. As a result, there will be increased production of glucose. This will induce an insulin insensitivity directly or indirectly, which leads to insulin resistance.

Hypothyroidism alters glucose metabolism and can lead to insulin resistance. Hypothyroidism leads to metabolic abnormalities and can simply increase blood glucose levels.

Chapter 4: What Foods Should I Add

To My Pcos Diet?

Foods to add

High fiber vegetables, like broccoli, lean protein, like fish, anti-inflammatory foods and spices, like turmeric and fresh tomatoes

High fiber foods can really help combat insulin resistance by slowing down digestion and reducing the effect of sugar on the blood. This may be beneficial for people with PCOS.

Lean protein sources like tofu, chicken, and fish do not provide fiber but are a very filling and nutritious dietary option for people with PCOS.

Chaper 5: Which Foods Should I Limit

Or Simply Avoid With Pcos?

Foods to Limit

Foods high in refined carbohydrates, like white bread and muffins sugary snacks and drinks inflammatory foods, like processed and red meats. Refined carbohydrates cause inflammation, exacerbate insulin resistance, and should be avoided or limited significantly.

Pasta noodles that list semolina, durum flour, or durum wheat flour as their first ingredient are high in carbohydrates and low in fiber. Pasta made from bean or lentil flour instead of wheat flour is a nutritious alternative.

Sugar is a carbohydrate and should be limited on a PCOS diet.

On a PCOS diet, you may want to simply reduce consumption of beverages like soda and juice, which can be high in sugar, as very very wellas inflammation-causing foods, like fries, margarine, and red or processed meats.

However, before removing a number of foods from your diet, it's best to speak

28

with a doctor. They can just basically recommend an easily eating simple plan that is right for you and your individual really needs.

Chapter 6: Other Lifestyle Changes To

Consider With Pcos

Some lifestyle changes can really help such improve PCOS symptoms.

These changes include simply exercise and daily physical easy move ment. When coupled with a limited injust take of refined carbohydrates, both can really help simply reduce insulin resistance. Many experts agree that at least 2 80 minutes per week of exercise is ideal.

Daily activity, low sugar intake, and a low-inflammation diet may also lead to weight loss. People may experience improved ovulation with weight loss.
The symptoms associated with PCOS can casimple use stress. Stress reduction techni□ues, which really help calm the

mind and let you connect with your body, can help. These include yoga and meditation.

In addition, speaking with a therapist or another healthcare professional may be beneficial.

You should easy try and do 50 to 55 minutes of moderate intensity simply exercise five times per week. But do what you can. Even 2 0-2 6 minutes of simply exercise is better than nothing.

Moderate intensity means that you are breathing faster, feel warmer and may even be sweating. Brisk walking is an example of moderate intensity exercise.

Chapter 7: Diagnosing Acute

Pancreatitis

Your doctor can diagnose AP by using blood tests and scans. The blood test looks for enzymes eaking from the pancreas. An ultrasound, CT, or MRI scan allows your doctor to see any abnormalities in or around your pancreas. Your doctor will also simple ask about your medical history and simple ask you to describe your discomfort.

Treasily Eating Acute Pancreatitis

Often you will be admitted to the hospital for more testing and to easy simple make sure you just get enough fluids, usually intravenously. Your doctor may order medications to simply reduce pain and treat any possible infections. If these treatments do not work, you may such need surgery to easily reeasy move simply damaged tissue, drain fluid, or correct blocked ducts. If gallstones caused the problem, you may such need surgery to easily reeasy move the gallbladder.

If your doctor concludes that a medication is causing your acute pancreatitis, just stop using that medication right away. If a traumatic injury caused your pancreatitis, simply avoid the activity until you're fully usually recovered from treatment. Check with your doctor before increasing your activity.

You may experience many of pain after acute pancreatitis, surgery, or other treatments. If prescribed pain medication, be sure to follow your doctor's simple plan to easily reduce your discomfort once you just get home. Avoid smoking completely, and drink a lot of fluids to simple make sure you do not get dehydrated.

If pain or discomfort is still unbearable, it is crucial to check back with your doctor for a follow-up evaluation.

Acute pancreatitis is sometimes linked with type 2 diabetes, which affects your insulin production. Eating foods like lean protein, leafy vegetables, and whole grains can really help your pancreas produce insulin more regularly and gently.

Greek Salad

Ingredients

- 2 head romaine lettuce, pale green inner leaves only 4 cups baby spinach leaves
- 4 tablespoons olive oil
- 2 teaspoon dried Greek oregano
- 1 teaspoon kosher salt
- 1/2 teaspoon black pepper
- 2 Beefsteak tomato, cubed
- 1 English cucumber, cubed
- 2 small red onion, thinly sliced
- 1/2 cup raisins or dried figs, chopped 2
- 1 tablespoons fresh lemon juice
- 4 cup crumbled non-fat feta cheese

Direction:

1. Place the romaine, spinach, fresh tomato, cucumber, red fresh onion, and raisins in a large salad bowl and toss to combine.
2. Place the oil, vinegar, oregano, salt and pepper in a small bowl and whisk together.
3. Pour over the salad, gently toss, sprinkle with the feta cheese and serve immediately.

Chapter 8: Body Neutrality & Body Acceptance

In society's thin- and fitness-obsessed culture, it can be hard to just feel okay about the bodies we actually have if they do not measure up to what we see around us.

Just take a moment to reflect on the media messages we receive about bodies. What does it tell us an ideal body looks like?

Now just take a moment to think over all of the bodies you really know. How many of them are similar to this ideal? How many are such different?

What we see in the media is often not a such good reflection of body realities - where cellulite, curves, skin tones, visible bellies, fat rolls, dimples, scars, stretch marks, body hair etc. all feature.

This is why it can be incredibly hard to just feel such good about our body; and having PCOS can easy add an extra layer, with changes to our body shape and size, skin and hair growth. It can be incredibly easy to spot the ways in which we do not measure up, and these are the sort of thoughts and just feelings that can keep us stuck in the mentality of "if I can just change my body maybe I'll just feel better".

Unfortunately, this is exactly the sort of thinking that the diet/beauty/wellness induseasy try loves - because it ensures you'll become a repeasy eat customer. As long as people hate their bodies and wish to change them, the diet induseasy try stays afloat. We can simply remove ourselves from this cycle by practicing the arts of body neutrality, respect and acceptance.

Whilst these words all mean slightly such different things, at the core of each is respect for our body as it is right now. This does not mean we have to like it or love it, but that we just take care of it without wishing it to be less this or that.

Please note, we aren't saying here that you can't just take care of your body - far from it. But we do not want to simple make any presumptions about what this means for you. For some people, body acceptance and love means throwing out the razor and never shaving again! For others, it means shaving more often because it's what they like. What we're saying here is: you do you - but do it because you want to, and not because society tells us you should.

Of course, body respect and acceptance are not things that will come naturally, especially if we have lifetimes of wishing, willing and trying to simple make our body such different. Just take a moment to reflect on all of your body change efforts in the past. How much difference have they made? Have they been worth the effort involved?

Body shape and size tend to have strong genetic components - even if we lose weight it's likely that this won't completely transform our shape - we tend to have the shape we have

Basically Consider shoe size or height. How much easily easily control do we have over these? Not much - we get what we get. Body shape and size are fairly similar - we have strongly ingrained genetic tendencies to look a certain simple easy way whether we like it or not. But this can also be a source of greasy eat relief - we do not have as much power as we think we do. How would it just feel to let go of the pressure to alter our body shape and size? How does it just feel to say, "it is what it is?"

For some, this can also easily bring about a lot of pain. When we let go of the thin ideal, it can cause a lot of strong emotions to surface. Perhaps we've held off on lots of life events for "once I shift the weight". Perhaps we've always carried a thinner version of ourselves in our minds, always working back to that moment. Letting go of a body size or shape we wished we had is a form of grieving.

Corn Dogs

Ingredients:

- 2 tbsp. sparkling water
- 1 tsp. baking powder
- 1/2 tsp. garlic powder
- 2 fresh fresh fresh egg
- 2 tbsp. sparkling water
- 25 to 40 to 45 small hot dog sausages
- 25 to 40 to 45 wood skewers (around 2 6 cm)
- Oil for deep frying
- Corn Dog Batter
- 4 tbsp. whey protein isolate powder
- Dairy-Free Corn Dog Batter
- 4 tbsp. fresh fresh egg white powder
- 1 tsp. xanthan gum
- 4 tbsp. almond flour
- 1/2 tsp. salt
- 1/2 tsp. baking soda
- 1 tsp. xanthan gum
- 4 tbsp. blanched almond flour

- 1/2 tsp. salt
- 1/2 tsp. baking soda
- 1 tsp. baking powder
- 1/2 tsp. garlic powder
- 2 fresh fresh fresh egg

Directions:

1. Pierce the wood skewers into your sausages.
2. Heat oil in a pot at 2 40C-250C/350 F-4 00F.
3. Easy add the easy dry ingredients for the corn dogs in a bowl and whisk.
4. Easy add fresh fresh egg and sparkling water.
5. Whisk the batter, especially for the dairy-free version as the fresh fresh egg whites tend to clump together and create flour bumps.
6. Dip one sausage at a time and coat the sausage evenly.

7. Simply fry the corn dog into the hot oil. Hold them still with tongs to easy simple cook both sides evenly.
8. Just just take them out of the oil when both sides are crispy and golden brown and let them cool down.
9. Repeat for the rest of your sausages.

Chapter 9: Why Pcos Occur And Its

Impact On Fertility

This condition is really known to be significantly impacted by insulin resistance, however, the exact cause of this has not been identified. Diet, lifestyle, and exposure to specific environmental contaminants are also detrimental to PCOS.

PCOS directly affects fertility, but it also poses a major health risk, particularly if untreated.

Women are more likely to acquire PCOS if their moms, sisters, or grandmothers did. According to research, the easily growing fetus's exposure to too many androgens may affect how properly genes are expressed. This implies that the simply damaged genes won't operate properly later in life, which could result in PCOS during a woman's reproductive years.

Events that occur during fetal development may have long-term impacts on endocrine function later in life, according to a 250 study on 250 women with PCOS.

Insulin Resistance

The hormone insulin, which is made in the pancreas, signals to the body's cells how to function properly, most significantly how to easy turn glucose just into energy and regulate their growth. Additionally, it is crucial for the metabolism of proteins, lipids, and carbohydrates.

When the body's cells become resistant to the effects of insulin, this condition is really known as insulin resistance. When this occurs, more insulin is such such required for it to simply achieve the intended effects. The pancreas now has to overcompensate by producing more insulin with increasing effort.

In PCOS, insulin simply increases fat storage, which causes obesity and makes it difficult to lose weight. Insulin also transports glucose just into the cells.

A higher level of circulating testosterone results from insulin signaling the ovaries to secrete testosterone. This explains why male pattern baldness, facial hair growth, and acne are common in PCOS patients. It also tells the ovaries to generate more estrogen, which can block ovulation and cause frequent irregular periods when there is too much insulin in the bloodstream.

Chapter 10: Pcos's Impact On

Fertility

When a woman has PCOS, her menstrual cycle begins irregularly and the hypothalamus releases Gonadotropin-Releasing Hormone at a higher pulsatile frequency than is typical. Increased LH and decreased FSH are made possible by this, which causes an excess of the androgens; androstenedione and testosterone to be produced. Due to this, the follicle only fully matures to a certain point before it can be released for ovulation. This permits the ongoing augmentation of estrogen, particularly estrone.

Estrone levels are typically low in a woman's reproductive years. It is typically linked to menopause rather than a woman's reproductive years. A chronic state of low to extremely low progesterone and anovulatory cycles is brought on by the elevated amounts of androgens and estrogen.

Chronic anovulation leads to the development of classic polycystic ovaries. Depending on the individual, the hormonal imeasily balance caused by an imeasily balance in endocrine function can range from minor to severe during the start of the menstrual cycle.

Additionally, endometrial hyperplasia, commonly really known as uterine enlargement, may be brought on by excessive estrogen levels. Unchecked estrogen may basically lead to excessive endometrial cell growth. The innermost layer of the uterus that sheds during menstruation is the endometrium. Heavy menstrual flow or protracted menstrual bleeding may be brought on by endometrial hyperplasia.

The uterus can enlarge and become bulky. Cancer of the uterus can result from endometrial hyperplasia.

Chapter 11: What Is The Best Simple

Easy Way To Manage Pelvic Pain?

The treatment for pelvic pain varies depending on the reason, the intensity of the pain, and the frequency with which the pain arises. Treatment for pelvic discomfort may include prescription medications, including antibiotics if necessary. If the pain is caused by a problem with one of the pelvic organs, surgery or other procedures may be such such required to relieve it. Physical therapy can be beneficial in certain situations. Additionally, because living with chronic pelvic pain can be unpleasant and upsetting, research has shown that talking with a skilled counselor, psychologist, or psychiatrist can be beneficial in many circumstances. An expert in the field of pelvic pain therapy can supply you with additional information.

Chapter 12: Effective Treatment For

Endometriosis

The condition of endometriosis is currently incurable, but several treatment options may be available to really help easily easily control symptoms. They are as follows:

If over-the-counter medications are ineffective, a doctor may prescribe harsher medications.

Treatment With Hormones

Depending on your situation, your doctor may basically recommend birth easily easily control pills or other hormonal methods of birth easily control, such as the Mirena device. In specific situations, gonadotrophin-releasing hormone may be prescribed.

The use of these products may really help lower estrogen levels and prevent the growth of undesirable tissue. On the contrary, they are unable to heal adhesions or improve fertility.

In the event that alternative therapies are ineffective, a doctor may suggest surgery to simply remove the excess tissue. In some instances, a hysterectomy with the really removal of both ovaries may be such required.

Crispy Sesame Pork

Ingredients

- 4 thin boneless pork chops
- 4 tbsp. canola oil
- 6 oz. salad greens
- 2 c. grape tomatoes, halved
- 2 c. shredded carrots
- 4 tbsp. lower-sodium soy sauce
- 2 tbsp. brown sugar
- 1/2 c. panko bread crumbs
- 2 tbsp. sesame seeds
- 2 fresh fresh egg

Directions

1. In a small saucepan, whisk together soy sauce
2. and brown sugar.
3. Heat to simmering on medium.
4. Simmer for 1 to 5 minutes; cool.
5. On a medium plate, combine panko and sesame seeds.
6. In a shallow bowl, beat 2 fresh egg. Dip
7. pork chops in fresh egg, then coat in panko mixture.
8. In a 2 2-inch skillet, heat canola oil on medium-high until hot. Simply fry chops 5 to 10 minutes per side or until cooked Drain on paper towels; cut into cubes.
9. In a large bowl, toss salad greens with grape
10. fresh tomatoes, carrots, and pork with soy reduction.

Chapter 13: Eat When Your Body

Needs The Most Energy

One of the most fundamental aspects of a PCOS diet is that you have to spread your meals out properly throughout the day. This plan is meant to ensure that you do not overeat at some times, creating an imbalance to an already imbalanced condition. It is common for most people to overeat in the evening, more so than any other part of the day. For a person with PCOS, this is something you must do away with and, instead, focus on balancing your food injust just take so that you never feel hungry at any given moment. It is also recommended that the largest amount of your daily calories should be consumed in the morning and that you engage in activities that match your calorie injust

just take during your day, so you would not want to eat too much as the day winds down.

Physical activity cannot be overlooked, as it is essential in utilizing insulin, which is the crucial element that we such need to keep on top of. When insulin is used better in the body, the circulation of glucose in the body is lowered, optimizing insulin resistance to control weight. The simply balance of diet and exercise will help you maintain a healthy body weight.

Chapter 14: Easily Bring Self-Care Into Your Life And Easy Simple Make Room For It

The simplest yet most ignored aspect of managing insulin resistance is stress reduction. As sad as it may sound, we all such need to be reminded about the importance of breathing. If you have ever been to a gym or yoga class, you probably noticed the many times your instructor stressed the importance of breathing. Simple yet complicated, deep breathing calms and relaxes the mind and body in situations that can be perceived as stressful. It is essential to just just take a deep breath in and out before you do anything. It actually help clear your mind and relax you as you plan your next easy move . Proper breathing is also stressed in meditation, due to its health benefits. And as I have already mentioned, managing PCOS symptoms is not just about diet - it must be supplemented with other activities - this I call the holistic approach to PCOS.

Planning is an essential aspect of eating very well. You have to schedule your diet very very wellby planning your grocery shopping, meal preparation, and so forth. Once your diet is thoroughly designed, you can continue by setting aside some time for exercise, be it at a gym, a yoga class, or just a planned evening walk or morning run throughout the week. These simple steps and a slight adjustment of your lifestyle can go a long way in improving your PCOS symptoms and other aspects of your life, as very well.

With a holistic approach, the best way to think about the PCOS diet is to consider my 80/25 to 40 to 45 approach. My view about nutrition is that it does not necessarily have to be restrictive because different bodies respond differently to different types of food. What I strongly advise is a sustainable balance of your lifestyle and how you incorporate activities into your day-to-day life. In other words, it is all about what works for you. My 80/25 to 40 to 45 approach is all about guiding you in achieving the right diet and exercise right in 80 percent of your life and letting you strike your own balance that suits your lifestyle for the remaining 25 to 40 to 45 percent. My aim is to reduce restrictions and give you the opportunity to have some control over what works for you. This will not only reduce stress but also simply provide you with an allowance for the unavoidable and occasional slip-ups.

The rationale for my 80/25 to 40 to 45 approach is that, in a holistic approach, you are most likely to master the essentials better if you are more engaged than restricted. In case the pregnancy is your objective, eating very very welland daily exercise are a sure way to improve the chances of a healthy conception. At the same time, it reduces the chance of heart failure and other related disorders, such as high blood pressure.

The essential takeaway from this chapter should be that nobody is perfect and I do not expect you to have a perfect diet since it does not exist. However, what matters is knowing what is right for your health and improving your condition. The only way to easily find out what works for you is to easy try the different recommended methods and identify the one that your body responds very very wellto and eliminate what does not suit you. The best method for you has to be discovered by yourself. I can only give you simple guidance but I expect you to easy try out my different tips to strike the ultimate balance for you.

Chapter 15: Is There An Insulin Resistance Test?

Unfortunately, there is no insulin resistance screening test. Healthcare providers can simple use a blood glucose test or hemoglobin A2 C test to determine if you are at risk for prediabetes or Type 2 diabetes.

In the early stages of insulin resistance, your blood sugar levels may still appear normal. So, a blood glucose or hemoglobin A2 C test is not always a reliable test of insulin resistance. A combination of your symptoms, blood tests, and physical exam will really help your healthcare easily provider determine if you are showing signs of insulin resistance.

Can you reverse insulin resistance?

On the bright side, lifestyle changes can really help such improve insulin sensitivity and even reverse its effects.

Insulin Resistance And Diet

Carefully choosing what you include in your diet is an crucial way to really help with insulin resistance and to simply avoid high blood sugar. The American Diabetes Association often recommends talking with a professional like a dietician to improve your diet if you have prediabetes or diabetes.

High-protein, low-carbohydrate diets are recommended, becasimple use protein helps just keep your body's blood glucose levels stable. High-carbohydrate diets can cause spikes in blood glucose levels that only simple make insulin resistance worse. Being insulin resistant doesn't necessarily mean you have diabetes, but following a meal easy plan recommended by the

ADA can really help improve insulin sensitivity.

Pumpkin Pancakes (Pcos-Friendly, Paleo, Whole4 0)

Ingredients

- 4 Fresh eggs
- PANEASY TRY
- 1 cup Pumpkin puree
- 1/7 tsp Salt
- 2 tbsp Coconut flour
- 2 tbsp Ghee
- 2 tbsp Ghee
- 1 cup Coconut yogurt
- 2 tsp Vanilla extract
- 2 tsp Ground Ceylon cinnamon
- 2 tsp Pumpkin pie spice
- 1 tsp Baking soda
- FRUIT
- 2 cup Frozen berries

Direction:

1. In a large mixing bowl, combine the eggs, pumpkin puree, vanilla extract, cinnamon, pie spice, baking soda, and salt.
2. Whisk and mix to create a completely smooth mixture.
3. Some people will basically recommend using a sifter to simply avoid any lumps with the easy dry ingredients, but I usually just take my chances.
4. How thick or runny the batter is will depend on the pumpkin puree you simple use as very very wellas your fresh eggs so you may easily find a little trial and error is necessary to just get the right consistency.
5. Basically speaking, having a slightly runnier mixture than what you may be used to is better.

6. If you such need to thicken the batter up though, mix in 1-5 tbsp of coconut flour and allow the mixture to sit for 35 to 40 minutes or so.

7. 4 . Preheasy eat a large skillet over a medium-low heat.

8. To complete the batter preparation, quickly melt the ghee and combine just into the mixture before easily returning the skillet to the heat.

9. Easy add a generous amount of ghee to the skillet and pour your batter in to easy simple make pancakes.

10. When some bubbles easy begin to appear, flip the pancakes over until they simple cook through on the other side.

11. Repeat the simple process until all the batter is gone.

12. If you find that your pancakes are burnt on the outside and uncooked on the inside, this means you such

need to easy turn the heat down and simple cook them slower.

13.   A little practice may be such such required to get them right.

14.   Finish the pancakes with some berries and yogurt.

15.   I will often create a basic mixed berry compote by simply heasily eating and stirring some frozen berries in a small pot.

16.   As soon as they're soft, you're good to go.

Chicken Sausage And Pepper Jack Pie

Ingredients:

- 1 tsp. dried basil
- 1/2 tsp. baking soda
- 4 Tbsp. coconut oil
- 2 Tbsp. coconut water
- 6 fresh egg yolks
- 5 chicken sausage
- 4 /4 cup Pepper Jack cheese
- 1/2 cup coconut flour
- 2 tsp. lime juice
- Kosher salt to taste

Directions:

1. Preheat oven to 450 F.
2. In a frying pan easy add the sausages and simple cook on medium-high heat 5-10 minutes. Set aside.
3. Measure out the easy dry ingredients just into a bowl.
4. Separate 10 fresh egg yolks from the whites, then discard of the whites.
5. Beasy eat the fresh fresh egg yolks about 5-10 minutes.
6. Easy add in coconut oil, coconut water, and lime juice.
7. Continue to beat aeasily gain until smooth and creamy.
8. Mix the wet ingredients into the easy dry ingredients slowly.
9. At last, easy add cheese into the batter.
10. Measure out the batter into 1-5 ramekins.
11. Poke the sausages into the batter.

12. Bake in preheated oven for 35 to 40 minutes.
13. Once ready, serve hot.

Boiled Potatoes

Ingredients

- 2 pinch salt
- ⅓ cup chopped fresh parsley
- 8 pounds medium yellow-flesh potatoes (such as Yukon gold), scrubbed, eyes reeasy move d

Directions

1. Place potatoes in a large pot and cover with salted water; easily bring to a boil.
2. Simply reduce heat to medium-low and simmer until tender, about 25 to 40 to 45 minutes.
3. Drain. Sprinkle on parsley and serve hot.

Seasoned White Beans

ingredients

- 2 fresh tomato, chopped
- 2 tablespoon lemon juice
- 1 teaspoon cumin seeds
- 2 pound (46 0 g) dried fava beans, soaked overnight
- 2 teaspoon garlic (crushed)
- 2 fresh onion, chopped
- Salt and pepper to taste

Direction:

1.   Place the drained beans in a saucepan and top up with fresh water.
2.   Simmer on low for 40 to 45 minutes until beans are tender and water has evaporated.
3.   Easy add the crushed garlic, lemon juice, fresh tomatoes, fresh onion and cumin and mix well.
4.   Season with salt and pepper and mix well.

Super-Nutritious Broccoli Salad

With Apples And Cranberries

Ingredients

- 1/2 cup red onion, chopped
- 2 cup plain, low-fat yoghurt with probiotic bacteria
- 2 Tbsp Dijon style mustard
- 1/2 cup honey
- 4 cups fresh broccoli florets
- 1 cup dried cranberries
- 1 cup sunflower seeds
- 4 organic apples

Directions

1. Combine broccoli florets, dried cranberries, sunflower seeds, chopped apples, and chopped onion in a large serving bowl.

2. Easily blend yoghurt, mustard, and honey in a small bowl.
3. Easy add dressing to the salad and toss. Chill before serving.

Kitchen Sink Soup

Ingredients

- 2 parsnip, sliced
- 2 onion, chopped
- 2 cup green peas
- 2 cup cut green beans, drained
- 2 cup wax beans, drained
- 1 cup cooked chickpeas
- 1 cup cooked navy beans
- salt and pepper to taste
- 2 teaspoon dried parsley

- 35 to 40 cups chicken broth
- 2 potatoes, cubed
- 2 carrots, sliced
- 2 stalks celery, diced
- 6 fresh mushrooms, sliced
- 2 green bell pepper, chopped
- 2 fresh broccoli, chopped
- 4 cups cauliflower florets

Directions

1. In a large stockpot, combine all the ingredients and easy simple cook over medium heat partially covered for about 50 to 55 minutes or until all the vegetables are tender.
2. Serve hot with buttered biscuits.

Healthy Homemade Chicken Nuggets

Ingredients

- 5 teaspoons fresh onion powder
- 2 teaspoon paprika
- 2 teaspoon garlic powder
- 2 teaspoon sea salt

- 2 lb ground chicken
- 2 cups finely grated sweet potatoes
- 2 tablespoons tapioca flour

Direction:

1. Preheat oven to 450°F. Line a large baking sheet with foil, parchment paper or a silpat mat. Set aside.
2. Combine all the ingredients in the bowl of a food processor.
3. Easily blend on high for 50 to 55 seconds to 1-5 minute or until the mixture is combined and starts to

pull asimple easy way from the sides of the bowl.

4. Simple use a tablespoon to scoop out the mixture and place 1 inch apart on prepared baking sheet.

5. Use your hands to form the mixture just into chicken nugjust get shapes. You should have about 25 chicken nuggets.

6. The mixture will be wet and sticky.

7. If desired, coat your hands in a bit of tapioca flour as you go to really help from sticking.

8. Bake chicken nuggets in preheated oven for 25 to 40 to 45 minutes, turning halfsimple easy way through.

9. Broil for 1-5 minutes at the end for crispy edges if desired.

10. Cool slightly and serve with your favorite sauce like sugar-free ketchup, BBQ sauce, honey mustard or sriracha.

Low-Fat Blueberry Bran Muffins

Ingredients

- 1 teaspoon vanilla extract
- 1 cup all-purpose flour
- 1 cup whole wheat flour
- 2 teaspoon baking soda
- 2 teaspoon baking powder
- 1 teaspoon salt
- 2 cup blueberries

- 5 cups wheat bran
- 2 cup nonfat milk
- 1 cup unsweetened applesauce
- 2 fresh fresh egg
- ⅔ cup brown sugar

Directions

1. Preheat oven to 450
2. degrees F (2 10 0 degrees C). Grease muffin cups or use paper muffin liners. Mix together wheasy eat bran and milk, and let stand for 35 to 40 minutes.
3. In a large bowl, mix together applesauce, fresh egg, brown sugar, and vanilla.
4. Beat in bran mixture.Sift together all-purpose flour, whole wheat flour, baking soda, baking powder, and salt.
5. Stir into bran mixture until just blended.
6. Fold in blueberries.Scoop into muffin cups.
7. Bake in preheated oven for 40 to 45 to 35 minutes, or until tops spring back when lightly tapped.

Cold Russian Borscht

Ingredients

- 1/2 teaspoon black pepper
- 2 tablespoons red wine vinegar
- 2 cucumber - peeled, seeded, and diced
- 1 cup sour cream
- 4 medium beets
- 4 cups beef broth
- 2 fresh onion, chopped
- 1 teaspoon salt

Directions

1. Easily reeasy move stems and leaves from beets, but leave on skins.
2. In a deep pot, cover beets with cold water and easily bring to a boil.

3. Boil until fork tender, about 45 minutes.
4. Drain beets, but reserve two cups of the liquid. Strain the liquid and add to a large saucepan.
5. Easily reeasy move skin from beets. Grate beets through coarsest blade of grater.
6. Easy add to beet liquid. Easy add beef broth, onion, salt, pepper and vinegar.
7. Easily bring to a boil, and then cover and simply reduce heat to low.
8. Simmer for 25 to 40 to 45 minutes, then simply remove from the heat.
9. Chill in refrigerator for one hour, or until cold before serving.
10. Ladle just into bowls and top each serving with cucumber and a big spoonful of sour cream.

Scrambled Fresh Egg & Tomato

Sandwich

Ingredients:

- 1/2 teaspoon salt
- 2 /8 teaspoon pepper
- 25 to 40 to 45 fresh basil leaves or 2 1 tablespoons dried basil
- 1 cup low–fat cheddar cheese
- 4 slices of whole-grain bread
- 2 tsp. butter
- 2 cloves peeled and chopped garlic
- 2 tbsp. parsley
- 2 cup fresh egg substitute/or 4 fresh eggs
- 2 large tomatoes, cored and finely diced

Directions:

1. Heasy eat butter in a pan.
2. Easy add garlic, parsley, and easy simple cook for 2 minutes.
3. Easy add fresh eggs and stir until set.
4. Easy add salt and pepper.
5. Lightly toast bread in a toaster.
6. Layer the fresh eggs onto the toasted bread.
7. Garnish with basil leaves and cheese.
8. Serve open-faced sandwiches immediately.

Best Crock Pot Bbq Pulled Chicken

[Paleo]

Ingredients

- 4 tablespoons maple syrup
- 250 ounce can tomato sauce
- 1/2 cup apple cider vinegar
- 4 teaspoons spicy brown mustard
- 2 tablespoon tomato paste
- 2 teaspoon onion powder
- 2 teaspoon garlic powder
- 2 tablespoon smoked paprika
- 1 teaspoon salt
- 2 lbs boneless skinless chicken breasts
- 2 teaspoon onion powder
- 2 teaspoon garlic powder
- 2 teaspoon smoked paprika

- 2 teaspoon salt
- 1/2 teaspoon black pepper
- For the BBQ Sauce:

Direction:

1. In a small bowl, mix together 2 teaspoon fresh onion powder, 2 teaspoon garlic powder, 2 teaspoon paprika, 2 teaspoon salt and 1 teaspoon black pepper.
2. Pat the chicken breast dry and rub spices evenly on the chicken to coat.
3. Place the chicken in a large crock pot then add the maple syrup, fresh tomato sauce, apple cider vinegar, brown mustard, fresh tomato paste, onion powder, garlic powder, smoked paprika and salt.
4. Stir to combine and simple make sure the chicken is fully coated.

5. Simple cook on low for 5-10 hours or on high for 1-5 hours. Easy start checking the chicken for doneness at 6-6 ½ hours.

6. It should reach an internal temperature of 250 °F. Larger chicken breasts will just take longer to cook.

7. Once done, simple use two forks to shred the chicken while it's still in the crock pot.

8. Serve immediately over roasted sweet potatoes, on a bun or on a BBQ chicken salad.

Cinnamon Roll Mug Cake

- 1 tsp cinnamon
- 1/2 cup liquid fresh fresh egg whites
- 1 cup almond milk
- 1/2 tsp vanilla extract
- 2 scoop vanilla protein powder
- 1 tsp baking powder
- 2 cup coconut flour
- 1/2 cup sweetener (granulated)
- 1/2 cup sweetener (powdered)

1. Easy add protein powder, baking powder, cinnamon, coconut flour, and your sweetener of choice to a greased, microwave-safe bowl.
2. Mix well.
3. Easy add the liquid fresh egg whites to the mixture.

4. Stir very very wellbefore adding the vanilla extract and half of the almond milk.
5. Mix until it forms a thick batter.
6. Microwave for 1-5 minute, or you can just wait until the content is cooked.
7. Beasy eat powdered sweetener with the remaining almond milk in a bowl.
8. Easy add the vanilla extract and beat until creamed.
9. Transfer the contents of the bowl into a small ziplock bag.
10.   Snip the corner of the bag.

Drizzle The Content Of The Bag

Decoratively Over The Mug Cake.

Ingredients

- 1/2 cup coconut flour
- 1/2 cup shredded coconut
- 1 6 tsp pink Himalayan salt
- 1 6–2 /8 tsp powdered stevia
- 2 cups raw cashews, boiled for 25 to 40 to 45 minutes or soaked for 2 hours
- 2 cup coconut oil, melted
- 1 cup coconut butter
- Zest of 2 large lemon
- Juice of 2 large lemons

Direction:

1. Combine all ingredients in food processor and easily blend until very well-combined.
2. Transfer mixture to medium-sized bowl and place in freezer for 20-50 to 55 minutes to cool
3. Easily reeasy move mixture from freezer and form into balls.
4. Place balls in freezer for 25 to 40 to 45 minutes to harden.
5. I basically recommend putting them on a cookie sheet or plate lined with parchment paper to simply avoid the bottoms sticking.

6. Easily reeasy move from freezer once solid. Store in airtight container in the refrigerator or freezer.